54 Post Chemotherapy Juice Recipes:

Vitamin Rich Juices That Will Strengthen Your Body Naturally without the Use of Pills and Medicine

By

Joe Correa CSN

COPYRIGHT

This publication is designed to provide accurate and authoritative information in regard to the subject matter covered. It is sold with the understanding that neither the author nor the publisher is engaged in rendering medical advice. If medical advice or assistance is needed, consult with a doctor. This book is considered a guide and should not be used in any way detrimental to your health. Consult with a physician before starting this nutritional plan to make sure it's right for you.

ACKNOWLEDGEMENTS

This book is dedicated to my friends and family that have had mild or serious illnesses so that you may find a solution and make the necessary changes in your life.

54 Post Chemotherapy Juice Recipes:

Vitamin Rich Juices That Will Strengthen Your Body Naturally without the Use of Pills and Medicine

By

Joe Correa CSN

CONTENTS

ABOUT THE AUTHOR

After years of Research, I honestly believe in the positive effects that proper nutrition can have over the body and mind. My knowledge and experience has helped me live healthier throughout the years and which I have shared with family and friends. The more you know about eating and drinking healthier, the sooner you will want to change your life and eating habits.

Nutrition is a key part in the process of being healthy and living longer so get started today. The first step is the most important and the most significant.

INTRODUCTION

54 Post Chemotherapy Juice Recipes: Vitamin Rich Juices That Will Strengthen Your Body Naturally without the Use of Pills and Medicine

By Joe Correa CSN

The post chemotherapy period is extremely delicate and it varies from one person to another. Your cells usually recover with time but they need your help.

Some of the most common side-effects of chemotherapy are definitely nausea and vomiting, hair loss, weakness and fatigue, and weakened bone marrow.

There are lots of different medications that help reduce nausea, vomiting, and general weakness. But, instead of reaching for the pill each time you feel nauseous, you might try to help yourself in a more natural way. Doctors recommend drinking lots of fluids, often in small portions and what better fluid than a homemade juice that will load your body with plenty of nutrients for faster recovery. However, make sure to drink juice at least one hour before and after the meal, not with the meal.

Side effects are, unfortunately "normal" for this type of treatment. It is a way of your body telling you that it's weak and it needs help. This is why I have created a collection of post chemotherapy juices that are based on the world's healthiest foods full of key nutrients your body needs at this precise moment to heal and recover.

You went through an extremely difficult period in life and you deserve the best to regain your health and get back to your normal lifestyle. Try my recipes, maybe combine with some of your favorite ingredients and enjoy them every single day!

54 POST CHEMOTHERAPY JUICE RECIPES: VITAMIN RICH JUICES THAT WILL STRENGTHEN YOUR BODY NATURALLY WITHOUT THE USE OF PILLS AND MEDICINE

1.   Ginger Carrot Juice

Ingredients:

1 medium-sized carrot

1 medium-sized apple, cored

1 large cucumber

1 large beet, trimmed

1 small ginger knob, 1 inch

Preparation:

Wash the carrot and cucumber and cut into thick slices. Set aside.

Wash the apple and remove the core. Cut into bite-sized pieces and set aside.

Wash the beet and trim off the green parts. Cut into small pieces and set aside.

Peel the ginger root knob and set aside.

Now, combine carrot, apple, cucumber, beet, and ginger in a juicer and process until juiced.

Transfer to serving glasses and add some ice cubes and serve immediately.

Enjoy!

Nutrition information per serving: Kcal: 166, Protein: 4.7g, Carbs: 48.4g, Fats: 0.9g

2.　　Basil Honey Juice

Ingredients:

1 large artichoke heart

1 cup of avocado, cubed

1 large cucumber

1 cup of fresh basil

1 cup of green cabbage

1 tbsp of liquid honey

Preparation:

Using a sharp knife, trim off the outer leaves of the artichoke. Wash it and cut into small pieces. Set aside.

Peel the avocado and cut in half. Remove the pit and cut into cubes. Reserve the rest of the avocado for some other juice. Set aside.

Wash the cucumber and cut into thick slices. Set aside.

Wash the basil and cabbage thoroughly and torn with hands. Set aside.

Now, process artichoke, avocado, cucumber, basil, and cabbage in a juicer. Transfer to serving glasses and stir in the liquid honey.

Refrigerate for 30 minutes before serving.

Nutrition information per serving: Kcal: 357, Protein: 12.1g, Carbs: 63.6g, Fats: 22.8g

3.   Spinach Pomegranate Juice

Ingredients:

1 bunch of fresh spinach

1 cup of pomegranate seeds

1 cup of fresh kale

1 large lemon, peeled

1 cup of watercress

1 cup of Swiss chard

Preparation:

Combine spinach, kale, watercress, and Swiss chard in a colander. Wash thoroughly under cold running water. Drain and torn with hands. Set aside.

Cut the top of the pomegranate fruit using a sharp knife. Slice down to each of the white membranes inside of the fruit. Pop the seeds into a bowl and set aside.

Peel the lemon and cut lengthwise in half. Set aside.

Now, process spinach, kale, watercress, Swiss chard, pomegranate seeds, and lemon in a juicer.

Transfer to serving glasses and add few ice cubes before serving.

Enjoy!

Nutrition information per serving: Kcal: 357, Protein: 12.1g, Carbs: 63.6g, Fats: 22.8g

4.   Asparagus Pepper Juice

Ingredients:

2 cups of fresh asparagus, trimmed

1 large fennel bulb, trimmed

1 large green bell pepper, seeded

1 large yellow bell pepper, seeded

1 ginger root slice, 1-inch

2 oz of water

Preparation:

Wash the asparagus and trim off the woody ends. Cut into 1-inch pieces and set aside.

Wash the fennel bulb and trim off the wilted outer layers. Cut into small chunks and set aside.

Wash the bell peppers and cut in half. Remove the seeds and cut into small slices. Set aside.

Peel the ginger root slice and set aside.

Now, combine asparagus, fennel, green and yellow bell pepper, and ginger root in a juicer and process until juiced.

Transfer to serving glasses and stir in the water. Refrigerate for 10 minutes before serving and enjoy!

Nutrition information per serving: Kcal: 143, Protein: 12.1g, Carbs: 47.2g, Fats: 1.5g

5.   Honeydew Parsnip Juice

Ingredients:

1 large wedge of honeydew melon

1 cup of Brussels sprouts, trimmed

1 cup of parsnip, trimmed

1 cup of fresh broccoli

1 medium-sized apple, cored

2 oz of water

Preparation:

Cut the honeydew melon lengthwise in half. Scoop out the seeds using a spoon. Cut one large wedge and peel it. Cut into small chunks and place in a bowl. Wrap the rest of the melon in a plastic foil and refrigerate.

Wash the Brussels sprouts and trim off the outer leaves. Cut in half and set aside.

Wash the parsnips and cut into thick slices. Fill into the measuring cup and reserve the rest for some other juice. Set aside.

Wash the broccoli and chop into small pieces. Set aside.

Wash the apple and remove the core. Cut into bite-sized pieces and set aside.

Now, process honeydew melon, Brussels sprouts, parsnips, broccoli, and apple in a juicer.

Transfer to serving glasses and stir in the water. Add some ice and serve!

Nutrition information per serving: Kcal: 251, Protein: 8.7g, Carbs: 75.1g, Fats: 1.5g

6.　　Broccoli Mustard Greens Juice

Ingredients:

2 cups of fresh broccoli

1 cup of mustard greens

1 large grapefruit

1 cup of Romaine lettuce

1 medium-sized zucchini

2 oz of water

Preparation:

Wash the broccoli and chop into small pieces. Set aside.

Combine mustard greens and Romaine lettuce in a colander. Wash under cold running water and torn with hands. Set aside.

Peel the grapefruit and divide into wedges. Set aside.

Peel the zucchini and cut in half. Scrape out the seeds and cut into small chunks. Set aside.

Now, process broccoli, mustard greens, grapefruit, lettuce, and zucchini in a juicer. Transfer to serving glasses and add some ice.

Serve immediately.

Nutrition information per serving: Kcal: 166, Protein: 11.6g, Carbs: 48.6g, Fats: 2.1g

7.   Orange Cantaloupe Juice

Ingredients:

2 large oranges, peeled

1 cup of cantaloupe, cubed

2 medium-sized radishes, trimmed

1 ginger root knob, 1-inch

1 tbsp of liquid honey

2 oz of water

Preparation:

Peel the oranges and divide into wedges. Set aside.

Cut the cantaloupe in half. Scoop out the seeds and flesh. You will need about one large wedge for one cup. Cut and peel it. Chop into chunks and set aside. Reserve the rest of the cantaloupe in a refrigerator.

Wash the radishes and trim off the green parts. Cut into small pieces and set aside.

Peel the ginger root knob and set aside.

Now, process oranges, cantaloupe, radishes, and ginger in a juicer. Transfer to serving glasses and stir in the honey and water.

Add few ice cubes or refrigerate for 10 minutes before serving.

Nutrition information per serving: Kcal: 250, Protein: 4.9g, Carbs: 74.3g, Fats: 0.8g

8.　　Italian Tomato Juice

Ingredients:

2 large tomatoes

1 cup of fresh basil

1 cup of fresh celery, chopped

½ tsp of Himalayan salt

½ tsp of dried oregano, ground

Preparation:

Wash the tomatoes and place them in a bowl. Cut into quarters and reserve the juice while cutting. Set aside.

Combine basil and celery in a colander and wash under cold running water. Torn with hands and set aside.

Now, combine tomatoes, basil, and celery in a juicer and process until juiced.

Transfer to serving glasses and stir in the reserved tomato juice, salt. Sprinkle with some oregano for some extra taste.

Refrigerate for 10 minutes before serving.

Nutrition information per serving: Kcal: 64, Protein: 4.6g, Carbs: 17.8g, Fats: 1.1g

9.   Coconut Papaya Juice

Ingredients:

1 large papaya, seeded and peeled

2 large carrots

1 large lime, peeled

2 oz of coconut water

Preparation:

Peel the papaya and cut lengthwise in half. Scoop out the black seeds and flesh using a spoon. Cut into small chunks. Set aside.

Wash the carrots and cut into thick slices. Set aside.

Peel the lime and cut lengthwise in half. Set aside.

Now, combine papaya, carrots, and lime in a juicer and process until juiced.

Transfer to serving glasses and stir in the coconut water. Add few ice cubes or refrigerate before serving.

Enjoy!

Nutrition information per serving: Kcal: 347, Protein: 5.2g, Carbs: 119g, Fats: 2.4g

10. Yellow Juice

Ingredients:

1 large zucchini chunks

1 large lemon, peeled

1 cup of pumpkin

1 medium-sized yellow apple, cored

1 medium-sized banana

2 oz of water

Preparation:

Peel the zucchini and cut in half. Scrape out the seeds with a spoon. Cut into chunks and set aside.

Peel the lemon and cut lengthwise in half. Set aside.

Peel the pumpkin and cut in half. Scoop out the seeds using a spoon. Cut one large wedge and peel it. Cut into small chunks and set aside. Reserve the rest for later.

Wash the apple and remove the core. Cut into bite-sized pieces and set aside.

Peel the banana and cut into small chunks. Set aside.

Now, process zucchini, lemon, pumpkin, apple, and banana in a juicer. Transfer to serving glasses and stir in the water.

Add some ice and serve immediately.

Nutrition information per serving: Kcal: 254, Protein: 7.5g, Carbs: 72.9g, Fats: 1.9g

11.   Chia Juice

Ingredients:

1 large cucumber

1 large lemon, peeled

1 large lime, peeled

1 large orange, peeled

1 tbsp of chia seeds

2 oz of water

Preparation:

Wash the cucumber and cut into thick slices. Set aside.

Peel the lemon and lime and cut lengthwise in half. Set aside.

Peel the orange and divide into wedges. Set aside.

Now, combine cucumber, lemon, lime, and orange in a juicer and process until juiced.

Transfer to serving glasses and stir in some chia seeds for some extra nutrients.

Add few ice cubes and refrigerate for 20 minutes before serving.

Stir in the water after refrigerating and enjoy!

Nutrition information per serving: Kcal: 186, Protein: 6.2g, Carbs: 41.4g, Fats: 5g

12.   Swiss Chard Celery Juice

Ingredients:

1 cup of Swiss chards

1 cup of celery

1 medium-sized apple, cored

1 cup of collard greens

2 tbsp of fresh parsley

4-5 fresh spinach leaves

2 oz of water

Preparation:

Combine Swiss chards, collard greens, celery, and spinach in a colander. Wash thoroughly under cold running water and drain. Torn with hands and set aside.

Wash the apple and remove the core. Cut into bite-sized pieces and set aside.

Now, combine Swiss chards, celery, apple, collard greens, and spinach in a juicer and process until juiced.

Transfer to serving glasses and stir in the water. Add some ice and garnish with fresh parsley.

Enjoy!

Nutrition information per serving: Kcal: 106, Protein: 4.8g, Carbs: 31.3g, Fats: 1.1g

13.   Watermelon Watercress Juice

Ingredients:

1 cup of watermelon, seeded

1 cup of watercress

2 large leeks

1 large lemon, peeled

1 cup of beet greens

2 oz of water

Preparation:

Cut the watermelon lengthwise. For two cups, you will need about two large wedges. Peel and cut into chunks. Remove the seeds and set aside. Reserve the rest of the melon for some other juices.

Wash the watercress and beet greens thoroughly under cold running water and torn with hands. Set aside.

Wash the leeks and cut into 1-inch pieces. Set aside.

Peel the lemon and cut lengthwise in half. Set aside.

Now, combine watermelon, watercress, leeks, lemon, and beet greens in a juicer and process until juiced.

Transfer to serving glasses and stir in the water. Add some ice cubes and serve immediately.

Nutrition information per serving: Kcal: 156, Protein: 5.9g, Carbs: 44.2g, Fats: 1.1g

14.   Blueberry Butternut Squash Juice

Ingredients:

1 cup of blueberries

1 large orange, peeled

1 cup of butternut squash

1 medium-sized apple, cored

1 large kiwi, peeled

2 tbsp of fresh parsley

Preparation:

Place the blueberries in a colander and wash under cold running water. Drain and set aside.

Peel the orange and divide into wedges. Set aside.

Peel the butternut squash and remove the seeds using a spoon. Cut into small cubes and reserve the rest of the squash for some other recipe. Wrap in a plastic foil and refrigerate.

Wash the apple and remove the core. Cut into bite-sized pieces and set aside.

Peel the kiwi and cut lengthwise in half. Set aside.

Now, process blueberries, orange, butternut squash, apple, and kiwi in a juicer.

Transfer to serving glasses and garnish with parsley.

Refrigerate for 10 minutes before serving.

Nutrition information per serving: Kcal: 304, Protein: 5.9g, Carbs: 92.4g, Fats: 1.6g

15.   Strawberry Beet Juice

Ingredients:

1 cup of fresh strawberries

1 cup of beets, trimmed

1 large red apple, cored

1 large lime, peeled

1 ginger root knob, 1-inch

1 tbsp of liquid honey

2 oz of water

Preparation:

Place the strawberries in a colander and wash under cold running water. Drain and cut in half. Set aside.

Wash the beets and trim off the green parts. Cut into small pieces and fill the measuring cup. Reserve the beet greens for some other juice. Set aside.

Wash the apple and remove the core. Cut into bite-sized pieces. Set aside.

Peel the lime and cut lengthwise in half. Set aside.

Peel the ginger root knob and set aside.

Now, combine strawberries, beets, apple, and ginger in a juicer and process until juiced.

Transfer to serving glasses and stir in honey and water. Add some ice and serve immediately.

Nutrition information per serving: Kcal: 277, Protein: 4.2g, Carbs: 82.4g, Fats: 1.3g

16.   Sweet Potato Spinach Juice

Ingredients:

1 cup of sweet potatoes, cubed

1 bunch of fresh spinach

1 large cucumber

1 ginger root knob, 1-inch

Preparation:

Peel the sweet potatoes and cut into small cubes. Fill the measuring cup and reserve the rest for some other juice. Set aside.

Wash the spinach thoroughly under cold running water and torn with hands. Set aside.

Wash the cucumber and cut into thick slices. Set aside.

Peel the ginger root knob and set aside.

Now, combine sweet potatoes, spinach, cucumber and ginger root in a juicer and process until juiced.

Transfer to serving glasses stir in the water. Refrigerate for 15 minutes before serving.

Nutrition information per serving: Kcal: 190, Protein: 13.8g, Carbs: 51.1g, Fats: 1.7g

17.   Brussels Sprout Juice

Ingredients:

1 cup of Brussels sprouts, trimmed

1 cup of fresh broccoli

1 large artichoke head

1 large lemon, peeled

1 large cucumber

3 tbsp of fresh parsley

Preparation:

Wash the Brussels sprouts and trim off the outer layers. Cut in half and set aside.

Wash the broccoli and chop into small pieces. set aside.

Using a sharp knife, trim off the outer layers of the artichoke. Wash it and cut into bite-sized pieces. Set aside.

Peel the lemon and cut lengthwise in half. Set aside.

Wash the cucumber and cut into thick slices. Set aside.

Now, process Brussels sprouts, broccoli, artichoke, lemon, and cucumber in a juicer.

Transfer to serving glasses and garnish with fresh parsley. Refrigerate for 10 minutes before serving.

Enjoy!

Nutrition information per serving: Kcal: 140, Protein: 13.8g, Carbs: 48.1g, Fats: 1.4g

18. Green Bean Juice

Ingredients:

1 cup of green beans

1 cup of asparagus, trimmed

1 cup of fresh celery

1 large cucumber

1 cup of Romaine lettuce

1 large apple, cored

1 oz of water

Preparation:

Wash the green beans and cut into 1-inch pieces. Set aside.

Wash the asparagus and trim off the woody ends. Cut into small pieces and set aside.

Wash the celery and cut into bite-sized pieces. Set aside.

Wash the cucumber and cut into thick slices. Set aside.

Wash the lettuce thoroughly under cold running water. Drain and torn with hands. Set aside.

Wash the apple and remove the core. Cut into bite-sized pieces and set aside.

Now, process green beans, asparagus, celery, cucumber, lettuce and apple in a juicer. Transfer to serving glasses and stir in some water.

Add some ice and serve.

Nutrition information per serving: Kcal: 185, Protein: 8.1g, Carbs: 52.5g, Fats: 1.3g

19. Pumpkin Rosemary Juice

Ingredients:

1 cup of pumpkin, cubed

1 large yellow bell pepper, seeded

1 large orange, peeled

1 large lime, peeled

1 small rosemary sprig

Preparation:

Peel the pumpkin and cut in half. Scoop out the seeds using a spoon. Cut one large wedge and peel it. Cut into small chunks and fill the measuring cup. Reserve the rest for some other juice.

Wash the bell pepper and cut in half. Remove the seeds and cut into small slices. Set aside.

Peel the orange and divide into wedges. Set aside.

Peel the lime and cut lengthwise in half. Set aside.

Now, combine pumpkin, bell pepper, orange, and lime in a juicer and process until juiced. Transfer to serving glasses and sprinkle with some rosemary to taste.

Refrigerate for 15 minutes before serving.

Nutrition information per serving: Kcal: 149, Protein: 4.9g, Carbs: 44.6g, Fats: 0.7g

20. Mint Lime Juice

Ingredients:

1 cup of fresh mint

1 large lime, peeled

2 large honeydew melon wedges

1 large yellow apple, cored

2 oz of coconut water

Preparation:

Wash the mint thoroughly under cold running water. Drain and torn with hands. Set aside.

Peel the lime and cut lengthwise in half. Set aside.

Cut the honeydew melon lengthwise in half. Scoop out the seeds using a spoon. Cut two large wedges and peel them. Cut into small chunks and place in a bowl. Wrap the rest of the melon in a plastic foil and refrigerate.

Wash the apple and remove the core. Cut into bite-sized pieces and set aside.

Now, combine mint, lime, honeydew melon, and apple in a juicer. Transfer to serving glasses and stir in the coconut water.

Add some ice and serve immediately.

Nutrition information per serving: Kcal: 228, Protein: 3.4g, Carbs: 65.7g, Fats: 1g

21.   Grapefruit Raspberry Juice

Ingredients:

1 large grapefruit, peeled

1 cup of raspberries

1 large carrot

1 medium-sized apple, cored

1 small ginger root slice, 1-inch

1 oz of water

Preparation:

Peel the grapefruit and divide into wedges. Set aside.

Place the raspberries in a colander and wash under cold running water. Drain and set aside.

Wash the carrot and cut into thick slices. Set aside.

Wash the apple and remove the core. Cut into bite-sized pieces. Set aside.

Peel the ginger root and set aside.

Now, process grapefruit, raspberries, carrot, apple, and ginger in a juicer.

Transfer to serving glasses and stir in the water. Add few ice cubes or refrigerate before serving.

Enjoy!

Nutrition information per serving: Kcal: 239, Protein: 4.9g, Carbs: 76.2g, Fats: 1.7g

22.   Pineapple Cabbage Juice

Ingredients:

1 cup of pineapple chunks

1 cup of purple cabbage, chopped

1 large beet, trimmed

1 large carrot

A handful of fresh spinach

1 tbsp of liquid honey

Preparation:

Cut the top of a pineapple and peel it using a sharp knife. Cut into small chunks and fill the measuring cup. Reserve the rest of the pineapple in a refrigerator.

Wash the purple cabbage and spinach thoroughly torn with hands. Set aside.

Wash the beet and trim off the green parts. Cut into small pieces and set aside.

Wash the carrot and cut into thick slices. Set aside.

Now, process pineapple, cabbage, beet, carrot, and spinach in a juicer.

Transfer to serving glasses and stir in the liquid honey. Add few ice cubes and serve immediately.

Enjoy!

Nutrition information per serving: Kcal: 205, Protein: 5g, Carbs: 62.1g, Fats: 0.7g

23.   Fuji Juice

Ingredients:

2 medium-sized Fuji apples

1 large lemon, peeled

1 large cucumber

3 medium-sized celery stalks

A handful of spinach

2 oz of water

Preparation:

Wash the apples and remove the core. Cut into bite-sized pieces and set aside.

Peel the lemon and cut lengthwise in half. Set aside.

Wash the cucumber and cut into thick slices. Set aside.

Wash the celery stalks and cut into 1-inch pieces. Set aside.

Wash the spinach thoroughly and torn with hands. Set aside.

Now, process apples, lemon, cucumber, celery, and spinach in a juicer. Transfer to serving glasses and stir in the water.

Add some ice and serve.

Nutrition information per serving: Kcal: 224, Protein: 5.2g, Carbs: 65.4g, Fats: 1.5g

24.   Zucchini Pear Juice

Ingredients:

1 medium-sized zucchini

1 large pear, cored

1 cup of fresh broccoli, chopped

1 large fennel bulb

1 small ginger root slice

Preparation:

Peel the zucchini and cut in half. Scrape out the seeds with a spoon. Cut into chunks and set aside.

Wash the pear and remove the core. Cut into small pieces and set aside.

Wash the broccoli and cut into small pieces and set aside.

Trim off the outer leaves of the artichoke using a sharp knife. Cut into small pieces and set aside.

Peel the ginger root and set aside.

Now, process zucchini, pear, broccoli, fennel, and ginger in a juicer.

Transfer to serving glasses and add some ice before serving.

Nutrition information per serving: Kcal: 195, Protein: 8.7g, Carbs: 64.5g, Fats: 1.8g

25.   Parsley Juice

Ingredients:

1 cup of fresh parsley, torn

2 cups of Swiss chard

1 large cucumber

1 small yellow apple, cored

1 small orange, peeled

Preparation:

Combine parsley and Swiss chard in a colander and wash thoroughly under cold running water. Drain and torn with hands. Set aside.

Wash the cucumber and cut into thick slices. Set aside.

Wash the apple and remove the core. Cut into bite-sized pieces and set aside.

Peel the orange and divide into wedges. Set aside.

Now, combine parsley, Swiss chard, cucumber apple, and orange in a juicer and process until juiced. Transfer to serving glasses and add some ice before serving.

Enjoy!

Nutrition information per serving: Kcal: 161, Protein: 6.3g, Carbs: 46.3g, Fats: 1.2g

26.   Jalapeno Watermelon Juice

Ingredients:

2 cups of watermelon, seeded

1 cup of Romaine lettuce, chopped

1 large orange, peeled

1 cup of fresh basil, chopped

¼ tsp of jalapeno pepper, ground

Preparation:

Cut the watermelon lengthwise. For two cups, you will need about two large wedges. Peel and cut into chunks. Remove the seeds and set aside. Reserve the rest of the melon for some other juices.

Combine lettuce and basil in a colander and wash under cold running water. Drain and chop into small pieces. Set aside.

Peel the orange and divide into wedges. Set aside.

Now, process watermelon, lettuce, basil, and orange in a juicer.

Transfer to serving glasses and stir in the jalapeno pepper for some extra spicy flavor. Refrigerate for 15 minutes before serving.

Enjoy!

Nutrition information per serving: Kcal: 165, Protein: 4.9g, Carbs: 46.7g, Fats: 1g

27.   Arugula Juice

Ingredients:

1 cup of fresh arugula

1 cup of fresh mint

1 large carrot

1 large orange, peeled

1 large red bell pepper, seeded

Preparation:

Combine arugula and mint in a colander and wash thoroughly under cold running water. Drain and torn with hands. Set aside.

Wash the carrot and cut into thick slices. Set aside.

Peel the orange and divide into wedges. Set aside.

Wash the bell pepper and cut in half. Remove the seeds and chop into small slices. Set aside.

Now, combine arugula, mint, carrot, orange, and bell pepper in a juicer and process until juiced.

Transfer to serving glasses and stir in the water. You can add a pinch of Himalayan salt, but this is optional.

Add some ice and serve immediately.

Nutrition information per serving: Kcal: 153, Protein: 7.9g, Carbs: 47.3g, Fats: 1.3g

28.　Mixed Greens Juice

Ingredients:

1 cup of collard greens, chopped

1 cup of Swiss chard, chopped

1 cup of red leaf lettuce, chopped

1 cup of Romaine lettuce, chopped

1 large cucumber

1 large orange, peeled

1 large lemon, peeled

2 oz of water

Preparation:

Combine collard greens, Swiss chard, red leaf lettuce, and Romaine lettuce in a colander. Wash under cold running water and drain. Torn with hands and set aside.

Wash the cucumber and cut into thick slices. Set aside.

Peel the orange and divide into wedges. Set aside.

Peel the lemon and cut lengthwise in half. Set aside.

Now, process collard greens, Swiss chard, red leaf lettuce, Romaine lettuce, cucumber, orange, and lemon in a juicer.

Transfer to serving glasses and stir in the water.

Add some ice and serve immediately.

Nutrition information per serving: Kcal: 136, Protein: 7g, Carbs: 43.4g, Fats: 1.2g

29.   Broccoli Plum Juice

Ingredients:

5 large plums, pitted

1 cup of fresh broccoli

1 large cucumber

1 medium-sized apple, cored

Preparation:

Wash the plums and cut in half. Remove the pits and set aside.

Wash the broccoli and cut into small pieces. Set aside.

Wash the cucumber and cut into thick slices and set aside.

Wash the apple and remove the core. Cut into bite-sized pieces and set aside.

Now, combine plums, broccoli, cucumber, and apple in a juicer and process until juiced.

Transfer to serving glasses and add few ice cubes before serving.

Enjoy!

Nutrition information per serving: Kcal: 268, Protein: 7.6g, Carbs: 77.4g, Fats: 1.9g

30.   Sweet Apricot Juice

Ingredients:

1 cup of apricots, pitted and halved

1 large lemon, peeled

1 large carrot

1 medium-sized green apple, cored

1 tbsp of liquid honey

2 oz of water

Preparation:

Wash the apricots and cut in half. Remove the pits and fill the measuring cup. Reserve the rest for some other juice. Set aside.

Peel the lemon and cut lengthwise in half. Set aside.

Wash the carrot and cut into thick slices and set aside.

Wash the apple and remove the core. Cut into bite-sized pieces and set aside.

Now, combine apricots, lemon, carrot, and apple in a juicer and process until juiced.

Transfer to serving glasses and stir in the liquid honey and water.

Refrigerate for 15 minutes before serving.

Nutrition information per serving: Kcal: 243, Protein: 4.2g, Carbs: 69.3g, Fats: 1.3g

31. Mango Kale Juice

Ingredients:

1 cup of mango, chopped

1 cup of fresh kale

1 large artichoke head

1 large cucumber

1 ginger root knob, 1 inch

2 oz of water

Preparation:

Wash the mango and cut into small chunks. Fill the measuring cup and reserve the rest for some other juice. Set aside.

Wash the kale thoroughly and torn with hands. Set aside.

Wash the cucumber and cut into thick slices. Set aside.

Peel the ginger root knob and set aside.

Now, process mango, kale, cucumber, and ginger in a juicer.

Transfer to serving glasses and stir in the water. Add some ice and serve.

Enjoy!

Nutrition information per serving: Kcal: 197, Protein: 11.6g, Carbs: 59.6g, Fats: 1.8g

32.   Green Cayenne Juice

Ingredients:

1 cup of fresh broccoli

1 large carrot

1 large leek

1 cup of kale, chopped

1 large lime, peeled

1 large lemon, peeled

1 large cucumber

¼ tsp of Cayenne pepper, ground

Preparation:

Wash the broccoli and cut into small pieces and set aside.

Wash the carrot and cucumber and cut into thick slices. Set aside.

Wash the kale and celery thoroughly under cold running water. Roughly chop it and set aside.

Peel the lemon and lime and cut lengthwise in half. Set aside.

Now, process broccoli, carrot, kale, leek, lemon, and lime in a juicer.

Transfer to serving glasses and stir in the Cayenne pepper for extra spicy flavor.

Refrigerate for 30 minutes before serving.

Nutrition information per serving: Kcal: 174, Protein: 10.2g, Carbs: 51.4g, Fats: 1.9g

33.   Winter Squash Juice

Ingredients:

2 cups of butternut squash, seeded

2 large carrots

1 large Granny Smith Apple

1 small ginger root slice

Preparation:

Peel the butternut squash and remove the seeds using a spoon. Cut into small cubes and fill the measuring cup. Reserve the rest of the squash for some other juice. Wrap in a plastic foil and refrigerate.

Wash the carrots and cut into thick slices. Set aside.

Wash the apple and remove the core. Cut into bite-sized pieces and set aside.

Peel the ginger slice and set aside.

Now, process butternut squash, carrots, apple, and ginger in a juicer.

Transfer to serving glasses and refrigerate before serving.

Nutrition information per serving: Kcal: 246, Protein: 5.1g, Carbs: 75g, Fats: 1.1g

34. Radish Beet Juice

Ingredients:

1 large orange, peeled

1 cup of beets, trimmed and chopped

1 large radish, chopped

1 cup of fresh kale, chopped

1 large cucumber

Preparation:

Peel the orange and divide into wedges. Set aside.

Wash the beets and trim off the green parts. Chop into bite-sized pieces and set aside.

Wash the radish and trim off the green parts. Cut into small pieces and set aside.

Wash the kale thoroughly under cold running water. Drain and torn with hands. Set aside.

Wash the cucumber and cut into thick slices. Set aside.

Now, combine orange, beets, radish, kale, and cucumber in a juicer and process until juiced.

Transfer to serving glasses and add some ice before serving.

Enjoy!

Nutrition information per serving: Kcal: 174, Protein: 8.8g, Carbs: 51.7g, Fats: 1.4g

35.   Fennel Greens Juice

Ingredients:

1 large fennel bulb

1 large yellow apple, cored

1 cup of fresh kale, chopped

1 cup of mustard greens

1 large bell pepper, seeded

Preparation:

Wash the fennel bulb and trim off the wilted outer layers. Cut into small chunks and set aside.

Wash the apple and remove the core. Cut into bite-sized pieces and set aside.

Combine kale and mustard greens in a colander. Wash under cold running water and torn with hands. Set aside.

Wash the bell pepper and cut in half. Remove the seeds and chop into small slices. Set aside.

Now, process fennel, apple, kale, mustard greens, and bell pepper in a juicer.

Transfer to serving glasses and refrigerate for 10 minutes before serving.

Nutrition information per serving: Kcal: 199, Protein: 9.4g, Carbs: 62.4g, Fats: 1.9g

36.   Summer Peach Juice

Ingredients:

2 large peaches, pitted and halved

1 cup of apricots, pitted and halved

1 cup of cantaloupe, chopped

3 oz of coconut water

Preparation:

Wash the peaches and cut in half. Remove the pits and cut into bite-sized pieces. Set aside.

Wash the apricots and cut in half. Remove the pits and fill the measuring cup. Reserve the rest for some other juice. Set aside.

Cut the cantaloupe in half. Scoop out the seeds and cut about two large wedges. Peel and chop into chunks. Fill the measuring cup and reserve the rest of the cantaloupe in a refrigerator for some other juice.

Now, process peaches, apricots, and cantaloupe in a juicer.

Transfer to serving glasses and stir in the coconut water. Add some ice and serve immediately.

Enjoy!

Nutrition information per serving: Kcal: 239, Protein: 6.8g, Carbs: 66.4g, Fats: 1.8g

37.   Brussels Sprout Asparagus Juice

Ingredients:

1 cup of asparagus, trimmed

1 cup of Brussels sprouts, trimmed

1 large tomato

1 cup of Swiss chard

1 large cucumber

Preparation:

Wash the asparagus and trim off the woody ends. Cut into 1-inch pieces and set aside.

Wash the Brussels sprouts and trim off the outer layers. Cut in half and set aside.

Wash the tomato and place in a bowl. Cut into quarters and reserve the juice while cutting. Set aside.

Wash the Swiss chard thoroughly under cold running water. Drain and set aside.

Wash the cucumber and cut into thick slices. Set aside.

Now, process asparagus, Brussels sprouts, tomato, Swiss chard, and cucumber in a juicer.

Transfer to serving glasses and add some ice before serving.

Nutrition information per serving: Kcal: 109, Protein: 10.1g, Carbs: 32.4g, Fats: 1.2g

38.   Beets & Grapes Juice

Ingredients:

3 large beets, trimmed

2 cups of green grapes

1 cup of cauliflower, chopped

1 large lemon, peeled

Preparation:

Wash the beets and trim off the green parts. Cut into bite-sized pieces and set aside.

Wash the green grapes under cold running water. Set aside.

Trim off the outer leaves of cauliflower. Wash it and cut into small pieces. Fill the measuring cup and reserve the rest for some other juice. Set aside.

Peel the lemon and cut lengthwise in half. Set aside.

Now, process beets, grapes, cauliflower, and lemon in a juicer.

Transfer to serving glasses and add some ice cubes before serving.

Enjoy!

Nutrition information per serving: Kcal: 226, Protein: 7.8g, Carbs: 65.8g, Fats: 1.5g

39. Turnip Greens Juice

Ingredients:

1 cup of turnip greens, chopped

1 cup of kale, chopped

1 cup of Romaine lettuce, chopped

1 cup of cauliflower, chopped

1 large cucumber

Preparation:

Combine turnip greens, kale, and Romaine lettuce in a colander and wash under cold running water. Drain and roughly chop it. Set aside.

Trim off the outer leaves of cauliflower. Wash it and cut into small pieces. Fill the measuring cup and reserve the rest for some other juice. Set aside.

Wash the cucumber and cut into thick slices. Set aside.

Now, combine turnip greens, kale, Romaine lettuce, cauliflower, and cucumber in a juicer and process until juiced.

Transfer to serving glasses and add some ice before serving.

Enjoy!

Nutrition information per serving: Kcal: 96, Protein: 8.3g, Carbs: 27.6g, Fats: 1.6g

40.   Cranberry Apple Juice

Ingredients:

1 cup of cranberries

1 large red apple, cored

1 large lime, peeled

1 large orange, peeled

1 small ginger root knob, 1-inch

Preparation:

Place the cranberries in a colander and wash under cold running water. Drain and set aside.

Wash the apple and remove the core. Cut into bite-sized pieces and set aside.

Peel the lime and cut lengthwise in half. Set aside.

Peel the orange and divide into wedges. Set aside.

Peel the ginger knob and set aside.

Now, process cranberries, apple, lime, orange, and ginger in a juicer.

Transfer to serving glasses and refrigerate for 15 minutes before serving.

Enjoy!

Nutrition information per serving: Kcal: 240, Protein: 3.1g, Carbs: 75.1g, Fats: 0.9g

41.   Tomato Avocado Juice

Ingredients:

1 large tomato

1 cup of avocado, chopped

1 large cucumber

1 large lemon, peeled

1 cup of fresh basil, chopped

Preparation:

Wash the tomato and place in a bowl. Cut into quarters and reserve the juice while cutting. Set aside.

Peel the avocado and cut in half. Remove the pit and cut into chunks. Fill the measuring cup and reserve the rest for some other juice. Keep it in a refrigerator.

Wash the cucumber and cut into thick slices. Set aside.

Peel the lemon and cut lengthwise in half. Set aside.

Wash the basil thoroughly and roughly chop it. Set aside.

Now, combine tomato, avocado, cucumber, lemon and basil in a juicer and process until juiced.

Transfer to serving glasses and add some ice before serving.

Enjoy!

Nutrition information per serving: Kcal: 240, Protein: 3.1g, Carbs: 75.1g, Fats: 0.9g

42.   Parsnip Zucchini Juice

Ingredients:

1 cup of parsnips, chopped

1 large zucchini, seeded

1 cup of sweet potatoes, chopped

1 ginger root slice, 1-inch

2 oz of water

Preparation:

Wash the parsnips and trim off the green parts. Cut into thick slices and fill the measuring cup. Reserve the rest for some other juice.

Peel the zucchini and cut in half. Scrape out the seeds with a spoon. Cut into chunks and set aside.

Peel the sweet potato and cut into chunks. Fill the measuring cup and reserve the rest for some other juice. Set aside.

Peel the ginger root and set aside.

Now, process parsnips, zucchini, sweet potato, and ginger in a juicer.

Transfer to serving glasses and stir in the water.

Refrigerate for 10 minutes before serving.

Nutrition information per serving: Kcal: 216, Protein: 7.6g, Carbs: 61.1g, Fats: 1.5g

43.   Pomegranate Beets Juice

Ingredients:

1 cup of pomegranate seeds

1 cup of beets, trimmed and chopped

1 large lime, peeled

2 large carrots

1 large cucumber

Preparation:

Cut the top of the pomegranate fruit using a sharp knife. Slice down to each of the white membranes inside of the fruit. Pop the seeds into a measuring cup and set aside.

Wash the beets and trim off the green parts. Cut into bite-sized pieces and fill the measuring cup. Reserve the rest for some other juice.

Peel the lime and cut into lengthwise in half. Set aside.

Wash the carrot and cucumber and cut into thick slices. Set aside.

Now, process pomegranate seeds, beets, lime, carrots and cucumber in a juicer.

Transfer to serving glasses and stir in the water. Add some ice and serve!

Nutrition information per serving: Kcal: 194, Protein: 7.2g, Carbs: 57.7g, Fats: 1.9g

44.   Coconut Berry Juice

Ingredients:

1 cup of blackberries

1 cup of blueberries

1 cup of strawberries

1 cup of raspberries

1 cup of cranberries

3 oz of coconut water

Preparation:

Combine blackberries, blueberries, strawberries, raspberries, and cranberries in a colander. Wash under cold running water. Cut the strawberries in half and set aside.

Now, place all berries in a juicer and process until juiced.

Transfer to serving glasses and add some ice before serving.

Enjoy!

Nutrition information per serving: Kcal: 210, Protein: 5.9g, Carbs: 75.3g, Fats: 2.5g

45.   Watermelon Mint Juice

Ingredients:

1 cup of watermelon, chopped

1 large orange, peeled

1 large peach, pitted and halved

1 large Fuji apple, cored

3 tbsp of fresh mint, chopped

Preparation:

Cut the watermelon lengthwise. For two cups, you will need about two large wedges. Peel and cut into chunks. Remove the seeds and set aside. Reserve the rest of the melon for some other juices.

Peel the orange and divide into wedges. Set aside.

Wash the peach and cut in half. Remove the pit and cut into chunks. Set aside.

Wash the apple and remove the core. Cut into bite-sized pieces and set aside.

Now, combine watermelon, orange, peach, and apple in a juicer and process until juiced.

Transfer to serving glasses and garnish with some fresh mint. Add some ice cubes before serving.

Enjoy!

Nutrition information per serving: Kcal: 269, Protein: 5.3g, Carbs: 78.5g, Fats: 1.3g

46.   Plums & Beet Juice

Ingredients:

5 large plums, pitted and halved

1 cup of purple cabbage, torn

1 whole cucumber

1 large lemon, peeled

1 cup of beets, trimmed

2 oz of water

Preparation:

Wash the plums and cut in half. Remove the pits and cut into quarters. Set aside.

Wash the cabbage thoroughly under cold running water. Drain and torn with hands.

Wash the cucumber and cut into thick slices. Set aside.

Peel the lemon and cut lengthwise in half. Set aside.

Wash the beets and trim off the green parts. Cut into bite-sized pieces and set aside.

Now, process plums, cabbage, cucumber, lemon, and beets in a juicer.

Transfer to serving glasses and add some ice before serving.

Enjoy!

Nutrition information per serving: Kcal: 243, Protein: 8.3g, Carbs: 73.6g, Fats: 1.7g

47.   Avocado Juice

Ingredients:

1 cup of avocado, sliced

3 cups of red leaf lettuce, torn

1 large orange, peeled

½ cup of pure coconut water, unsweetened

1 tsp of liquid honey

Preparation:

Peel the avocado and cut in half. Remove the pit and chop into chunks. Fill the measuring cup and reserve the rest for some other juice. Set aside.

Wash the lettuce thoroughly under cold running water. Torn with hands and set aside.

Peel the orange and divide into wedges. Set aside.

Now, combine avocado, lettuce, and orange in a juicer and process until juiced.

Transfer to serving glasses and refrigerate for 10 minutes before serving.

Enjoy!

Nutrition information per serving: Kcal: 240, Protein: 4.9g, Carbs: 25.6g, Fats: 21.7g

48.   Mixed Berry Juice

Ingredients:

1 cup of blueberries

1 cup of strawberries

1 cup of cranberries

1 cup of raspberries

1 cup of blackberries

1 small granny Smith apple

¼ cup of water

1 tsp of pure coconut sugar

2 oz of water

Preparation:

Combine all berries in a colander and wash under cold running water. Cut the strawberries in half and set aside.

Soak the berries in water for 10 minutes. Drain and set aside.

Wash the apple and remove the core. Cut into bite-sized pieces and set aside.

Now, process all berries and apple in a juicer.

Transfer to serving glasses and stir in the coconut sugar and water.

Add some ice and serve!

Nutrition information per serving: Kcal: 210, Protein: 5.7g, Carbs: 82g, Fats: 2.4g

49. Orange Green Juice

Ingredients:

1 cup of broccoli, chopped

1 cup of Brussels sprouts, chopped

1 cup of carrots, sliced

1 cup of turnip greens, chopped

4 large oranges, peeled

1 tbsp of honey

¼ cup of pure coconut water

Preparation:

Wash the broccoli and cut into small pieces. Set aside.

Wash the Brussels sprouts and trim off the outer layers. Cut in half and set aside.

Wash the carrots and cut into thick slices. Set aside.

Wash the turnip greens thoroughly and torn with hands. Set aside.

Peel the oranges and divide into wedges. Set aside.

Now, combine broccoli, Brussels sprouts, carrots, turnip greens, and oranges in a juicer and process until juiced.

Transfer to serving glasses and stir in the honey and coconut water. Add some ice cubes before serving or refrigerate for 10 minutes.

Enjoy!

Nutrition information per serving: Kcal: 367, Protein: 14.47g, Carbs: 116g, Fats: 1.9g

50.   Fresh Apple and Cucumber Juice

Ingredients:

3 large Granny Smith apples, cored

1 large lemon, peeled

4 cups of cucumber

¼ cup of water

1 tbsp of liquid honey

Preparation:

Wash the apples and remove the core. Cut into bite-sized pieces and set aside.

Peel the lemon and cut lengthwise in half. Set aside.

Wash the cucumber and cut into thick slices. Set aside.

Now, combine apples, lemon and cucumber in a juicer and process until juiced. Transfer to serving glasses and stir in the water and liquid honey.

Garnish with some fresh mint, but this is optional.

Add few ice cubes before serving and enjoy!

Nutrition information per serving: Kcal: 327, Protein: 4.7g, Carbs: 97g, Fats: 1.5g

51.   Minty Apricot Juice

Ingredients:

5 apricots, sliced

1 large peach, sliced

1 large kiwi, peeled

A bunch of fresh spinach, chopped

1 tbsp of fresh mint, chopped

¼ cup of water

Preparation:

Wash the apricots and cut in half. Remove the pits and cut into chunks. Set aside.

Wash the peach and cut in half. Remove the pit and cut into small pieces. Set aside.

Peel the kiwi and cut lengthwise in half. Set aside.

Wash the spinach and mint under cold running water. Drain and roughly chop it. Set aside.

Now, combine apricots, peach, kiwi, spinach, and mint in a juicer and process until juiced.

Transfer to serving glasses and refrigerate before serving.

Nutrition information per serving: Kcal: 211, Protein: 2.8g, Carbs: 58.8g, Fats: 2.8g

52. Guava Ginger Juice

Ingredients:

1 large guava, chopped

1 ginger root slice, 1-inch

4 cups of Swiss chard, torn

4 cups of fresh kale, torn

A bunch of spinach, torn

¼ cup of pure coconut water, unsweetened

1 tbsp of pure coconut sugar

Preparation:

Wash the guava and cut into chunks. Set aside.

Peel the ginger slice and set aside.

Combine Swiss chard, kale, and spinach in a colander and wash thoroughly under cold running water. Drain and torn with hands. Set aside.

Now, combine guava, ginger, Swiss chard, kale, and spinach in a juicer and process until juiced.

Transfer to serving glasses and stir in the coconut water and pure coconut sugar.

Add some ice and serve immediately.

Nutrition information per serving: Kcal: 287, Protein: 30.8g, Carbs: 80g, Fats: 6.7g

53. Blackberry Watermelon Juice

Ingredients:

2 wedges of watermelon, seeded

1 cup of blackberries, fresh

1 large orange, peeled

½ cup of pure coconut water, unsweetened

1 tbsp of honey, raw

Preparation:

Cut the watermelon lengthwise. Cut two large wedges and peel them. Cut into chunks and remove the seeds. Set aside.

Wash the blackberries under cold running water and set aside.

Peel the orange and divide into wedges. Set aside.

Now, combine watermelon, blackberries, and orange in a juicer and process until juiced.

Transfer to serving glasses and stir the coconut water and honey.

Refrigerate for 10 minutes before serving.

Enjoy!

Nutrition information per serving: Kcal: 264, Protein: 7.2g, Carbs: 78.6g, Fats: 1.7g

54.   Raspberry Avocado Juice

Ingredients:

2 cups of fresh raspberries

1 cup of avocado, sliced

1 cup of kale, chopped

½ cup of pure coconut water, unsweetened

1 tsp of coconut sugar

Preparation:

Wash the raspberries under cold running water and set aside.

Peel the avocado and cut in half. Remove the pit and cut into chunks. Fill the measuring cup and reserve the rest for some other juice. Set aside.

Wash the kale thoroughly and torn with hands. Set aside.

Now, combine raspberries, avocado, and kale in a juicer and process until juiced.

Transfer to serving glasses and add some ice before serving.

Nutrition information per serving: Kcal: 351, Protein: 17.3g, Carbs: 65.2g, Fats: 25.4g

ADDITIONAL TITLES FROM THIS AUTHOR

70 Effective Meal Recipes to Prevent and Solve Being Overweight: Burn Fat Fast by Using Proper Dieting and Smart Nutrition

By

Joe Correa CSN

48 Acne Solving Meal Recipes: The Fast and Natural Path to Fixing Your Acne Problems in Less Than 10 Days!

By

Joe Correa CSN

41 Alzheimer's Preventing Meal Recipes: Reduce or Eliminate Your Alzheimer's Condition in 30 Days or Less!

By

Joe Correa CSN

70 Effective Breast Cancer Meal Recipes: Prevent and Fight Breast Cancer with Smart Nutrition and Powerful Foods

By

Joe Correa CSN

www.ingramcontent.com/pod-product-compliance
Lightning Source LLC
Chambersburg PA
CBHW051028030426
42336CB00015B/2772